FIRE SAFETY MANUAL

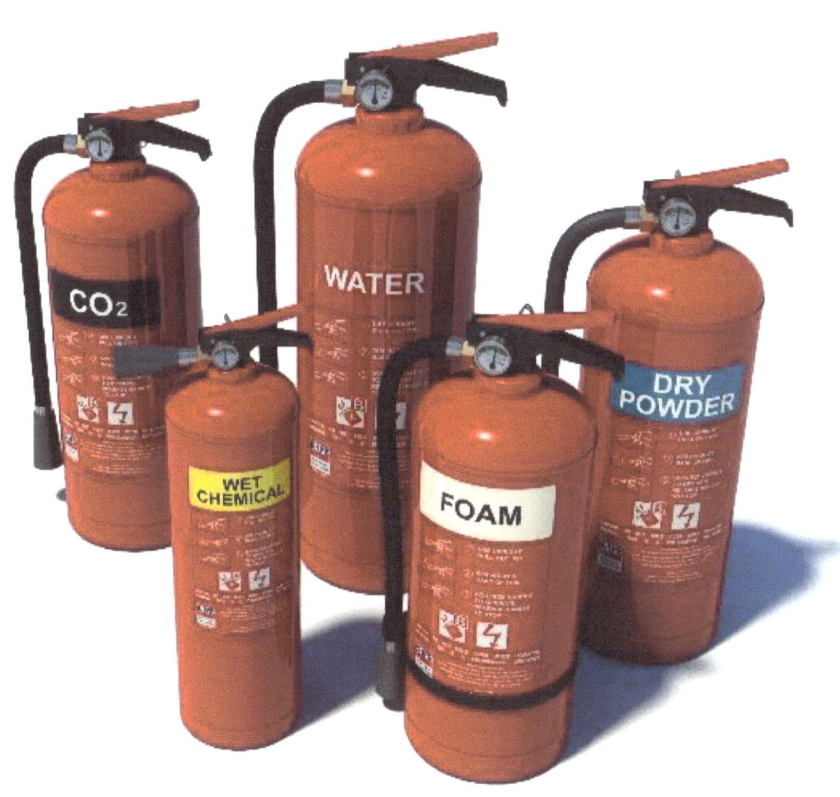

FAIRVIEW TRAINING

FIRST FOR TRAINING

© Blessing Isaackson 2024

All rights reserved. No part of this publication may be reproduced, stored in, or introduced into a retrieval system, or transmitted, in any form or by any means (electronic, mechanical, photocopying, recording or otherwise) without the prior written permission of the author of this book. The information presented in this book is accurate and current to the best of the authors' knowledge. The authors and publisher, however, make no guarantee as to, and assume no responsibility for, the correctness, sufficiency or completeness of such information or recommendation.

eBook ISBN: 978-1-7385781-2-2

Paperback ISBN: 978-1-7385781-3-9

Hardcover ISBN: 978-1-7385781-4-6

Table of Contents

INTRODUCTION 1

THE LAW 1

CAUSES OF FIRE IN THE WORKPLACE 3

THE FIRE TRIANGLE 4

HOW FIRE SPREAD 5

ACTION ON DISCOVERING A FIRE 5

EVACUATION PLAN 6

EVACUATING IN EMERGENCY 7

EVACUATION CHAIRS 8

CONSIDERATIONS BEFORE TACKLING THE FIRE 8

FINANCIAL COSTS 9

HUMAN COSTS OF FIRE 9

STEPS NECESSARY TO PREVENT FIRE IN THE WORKPLACE 9

CLASSES OF FIRE 11

FIRE EXTINGUISHERS 13

RISK ASSESSMENT 23

For fire risk assessments, there are five steps that you need to take: 24

Risk assessment 24

ROLE OF THE FIRE WARDEN 49

ROLE OF THE FIRE MARSHAL 49

BURNS AND BURNS KIT 55

INTRODUCTION

Each year, there are approximately 22,000 fires in the workplace in the UK, and 1,000 require hospital treatment.

On average, 350 people die every year in fire-related incidents.

20 people die on average in fire-related incidents in the workplace.

3200 people get injured in fire-related incidents.

About 60% of businesses fail within 2 years of a fire incident in the workplace.

THE LAW

Previous legislation governing the management of fire in the workplace

- Fire Precautions (Workplace) Regulations 1997
- The Fire Precautions Act 1971

Current law

The Regulatory Reform Order (RRO) (Fire Safety 2005): Replace all other fire safety regulations.

The Fire Safety (England) Regulations 2022 came into force on January 23, 2023.

- The new regulations will improve cooperation and coordination between responsible persons (RPs).
- Increase requirements in relation to the recording and sharing of fire safety information.

Make it easier for enforcement authorities to act against non-compliance.

Ensure residents have access to comprehensive information about fire safety in their building.

Other relevant legislation

Health and Safety Act 1974

Management of Health and Safety at Work Regulation 1999

Effects of the Regulatory Reform Order 2005

- Stopped the issuing of fire certificates.
- Fire certificates issued under previous fire safety laws are no longer effective.
- Makes provision for the appointment of a **"responsible person."**

WHO IS A RESPONSIBLE PERSON UNDER THE REGULATORY REFORM ORDER (FIRE SAFETY) 2005

You are the responsible person for fire safety if you are deemed to have control of the premises. For example, if you are an employer, The owner of the building. The responsible person needs eyes and ears on the ground.

- A fire marshal is an invaluable asset to keep a building and its occupants safe from fire.
- Good communication should be maintained between the responsible person and the fire marshals.

Role of the Responsible Person

- Provide a risk assessment.
- Carry out the fire safety improvements indicated in the risk assessment.
- Inspect existing fire safety measures.
- Maintain a fire logbook.
- Fire safety measures are to be maintained.
- Employees are to be trained regularly on fire safety measures.

CAUSES OF FIRE IN THE WORKPLACE

Arson and vandalism

- This accounts for about 35% of fires.
- Usually, employees or past employees.
- **Electrical faults and misuse**
- Plug in multiple blocks.
- Extension leads.
- **Smoking**
- Reduced by no-smoking policies.
- Disposing of cigarette ends in metal bins.
- **Heating Equipment: Portable and Fixed**
- **Flammable liquids and solids**
- **Unsafe storage**
- **Petroleum, oil, and lubricants**
- **Hot Work activities**

Contractors carrying out hot work activities should have the right fire extinguishers.

THE FIRE TRIANGLE

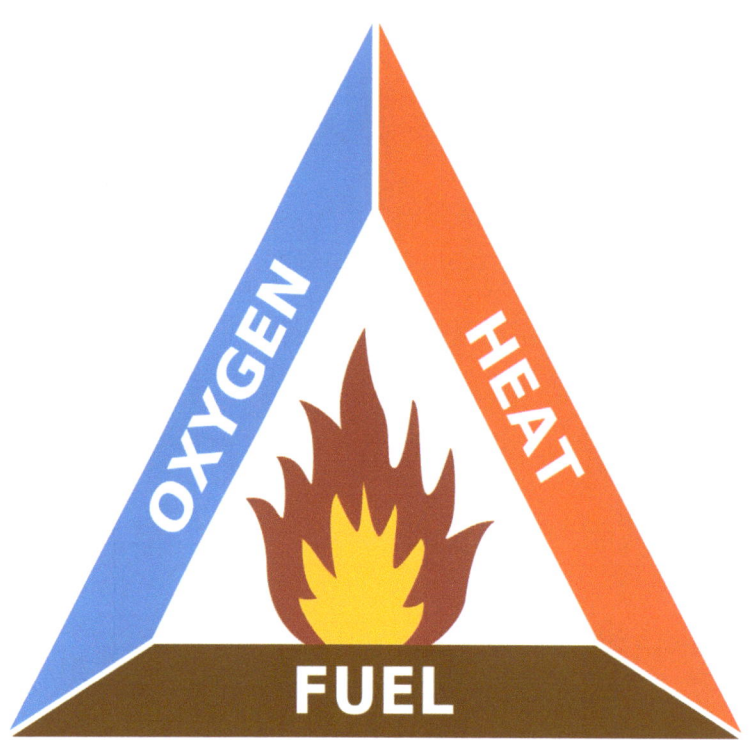

HEAT/Flammable materials + Fuel + Oxygen = Fire

(If you cool a fire, the fire will die.)

Heat can be started by:

- Cigarette
- Naked Flame
- Spark
- Friction

FUEL (a substance that will burn) + heat + oxygen = Fire (examples of fuel are wood, paper, and plastic). If the fire is **starved of fuel,** it will burn out. (Starvation is when the fire is deprived of fuel.)

OXYGEN: fire will die without oxygen. Heat + Fuel in the absence of oxygen = no fire (If the fire is deprived of oxygen, the fire will die. **This is called smothering.**

Fire requires all three elements of the fire triangle to exist. If you remove one of the elements, the fire will be extinguished.

Cool the heat, starve it of fuel, and smother the oxygen, and you kill the fire.

HOW FIRE SPREAD

CONDUCTION

Conduction is the transfer of heat within the material itself. Metal is a good conductor of heat.

CONVECTION

This is the transfer of heat by the physical movement of hot masses of air. That's why the air near the ceiling of a heated room is warmer than that near the floor.

RADIATION

This refers to the emission of energy in rays or waves. For example- Heat one feels sitting in front of a fireplace.

ACTION ON DISCOVERING A FIRE

- Shout "Fire, Fire, Fire" – alert as many people as possible.
- Close the door on the fire and, if possible, any windows, smoke can affect people on the upper floors, and the fire can spread.
- Sound the fire alarm – (break glass call point).
- Telephone the emergency services at 999 or 112, giving as much information as possible.
- **Attempt to fight the fire if you have been trained and it is safe to do so.**
- **Evacuate the building.**
- **Proceed to the assembly point for a roll call.**
- **Do not re-enter the building for any reason.**
- Shut Down Processes/Switch off Equipment-

1. Any processes or equipment that will escalate the fire;

2. or could endanger firefighters entering the building.

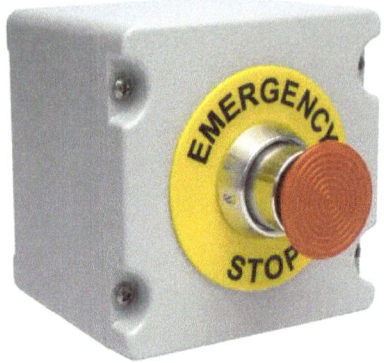 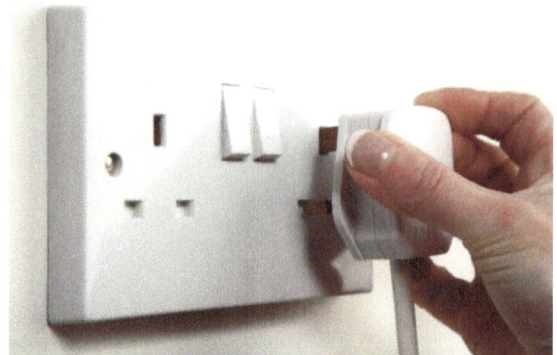

- Leave Premises Closing Doors

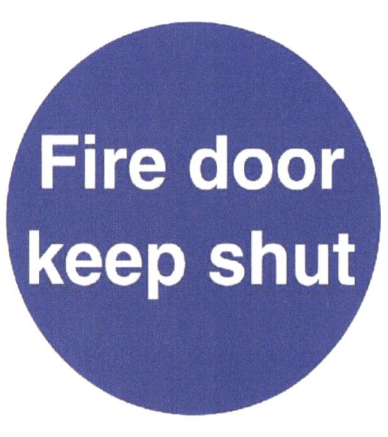 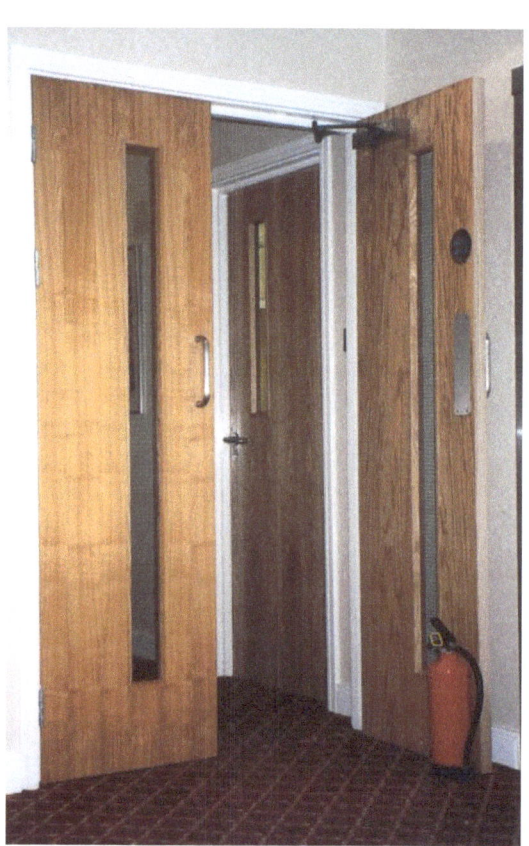

EVACUATION PLAN

- All buildings should have one. An evacuation plan should have the following:
- It must show you have a clear passageway to escape routes.
- Escape routes are marked as short and direct as possible.

- Enough exits and routes for all people to escape.
- Emergency doors that are open.
- Emergency lighting is available where needed.
- Training for employees to use the escape routes.
- A safe meeting point for all staff.
- Ensure everyone is aware of the evacuation plan and that it is tested and amended regularly.

EVACUATING IN EMERGENCY

- Evacuation procedures vary from workplace to workplace, Always follow the evacuation policies of where you work.
- Some workplaces have a stay-where-you-are policy.
- Care homes generally have a horizontal evacuation policy where you move to an exit but not downstairs.
- When you hear the fire alarm, do not panic, don't run, and don't carry your possessions.
- Follow the instructions from the fire warden/Fire Marshal.
- Once out of the building, head for the fire assembly point, where a roll call will be made to make sure everyone is out of the building safely.

WHAT WILL AFFECT THE ESCAPE OF OCCUPANTS
- Age
- Mobility
- Mental state
- Sight
- infirmity

EVACUATION CHAIRS

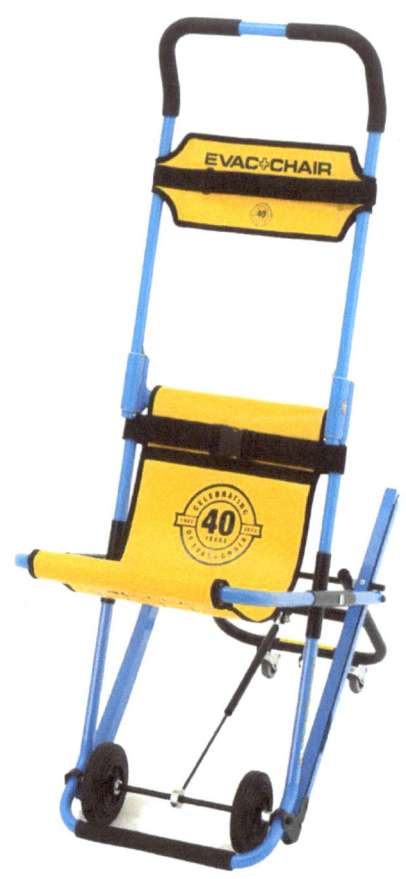

- Your role as a Fire Marshal is to evacuate everyone safely in the event of a fire.
- Special arrangement is required for those with mobility needs.
- Evacuation chairs help to transfer people with mobility needs.
- They are mounted on the chairs and ready to use.
- A person with mobility needs is strapped to the chair and helped to move down the stairs.

CONSIDERATIONS BEFORE TACKLING THE FIRE

- Is it within your capability?
- Do you have the correct extinguisher?
- Test the extinguisher before you use it.

- Do you have an escape route?
- If you don't put it out with one extinguisher, get out.
- If you are in any doubt about your safety at any time,

GET OUT AND STAY OUT.

FINANCIAL COSTS

- Staff absence - staff may be put off coming to work, and they might not be able to return to work, depending on the extent of the damage to the workplace.
- Damage to the building - the cost of assessing a building damaged by fire could be very high.
- Equipment damage.
- Damage to documents.
- Loss of morale.

Hefty fines can be imposed on businesses in breach of fire safety.

HUMAN COSTS OF FIRE

On average, per year

- 350 people die of fire-related incidents in the UK.
- 20 people die in work-related fires.
- There are 3,200 fire-related injuries.
- 20,000 workplace fires occur, and 1,000 require hospital treatment.

STEPS NECESSARY TO PREVENT FIRE IN THE WORKPLACE

- Keep sources of ignition and flammable substances apart.
- Avoid accidental fires.
- Avoid rubbish that can burn.
- Have the right firefighting equipment that puts out the fire quickly.

- Keep fire exits and escape routes clearly marked out.
- Train workers on procedures they need to follow to prevent fires in the workplace- fire drills.
- Risk assessment.
- Maintenance and testing of fire warning systems.
- Maintenance and inspection of firefighting equipment.

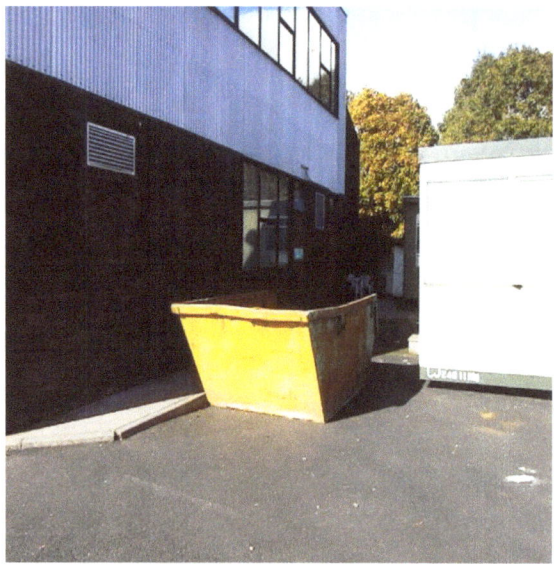

Skips

- 10 meters from buildings.
- Use enclosed rather than open.
- Arrange for collection as soon as it is full.

Staff Training

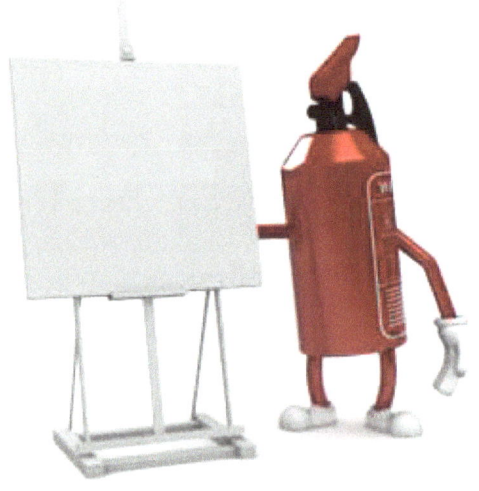

- Fire Awareness Training
- Induction training
- Fire Marshal training

CLASSES OF FIRE

Class A (Solid)

- Wood
- Paper
- Textiles
- Plastic

Class B (Liquids/Liquefied solids)

- Fuels
- Oils

Class C (Gas)

- Butane
- Propane
- Natural gas
- LPG

Class D (Metals)

- Metals
- Metallic powders

Electrical fires

Class F (Oils, Fat)

- Cooking Oils
- Fats

RULES WHEN USING THE FIRE EXTINGUISHER.

Remember **PASS**

P- Pull the pin

A- Aim low

S- Squeeze the handle

S- Sweep from side to side

- Only fight fires within your abilities.
- Fight the fire with the correct fire extinguisher.
- Test the extinguisher before approaching the fire.
- Always have your back to the escape route when fighting a fire.
- Keep the escape route clear.
- Avoid spreading the fire with the blast from the extinguisher.
- Use a colleague as a number two to provide extra support in case the fire worsens.
- If you do not extinguish the fire with the first fire extinguisher, consider the fire beyond your means. Get out, closing all the doors behind you.
- **If in doubt, get out and stay out.**
- Always call the fire brigade, even if you successfully put out the fire- they are the experts.

FIRE EXTINGUISHERS

➢ A minimum of 95% of the body of the fire extinguisher must be red. 5% of the body must denote the colour code of the fire extinguisher.

➢ The fire extinguisher must comply with BS EN 3.

WATER FIRE EXTINGUISHERS

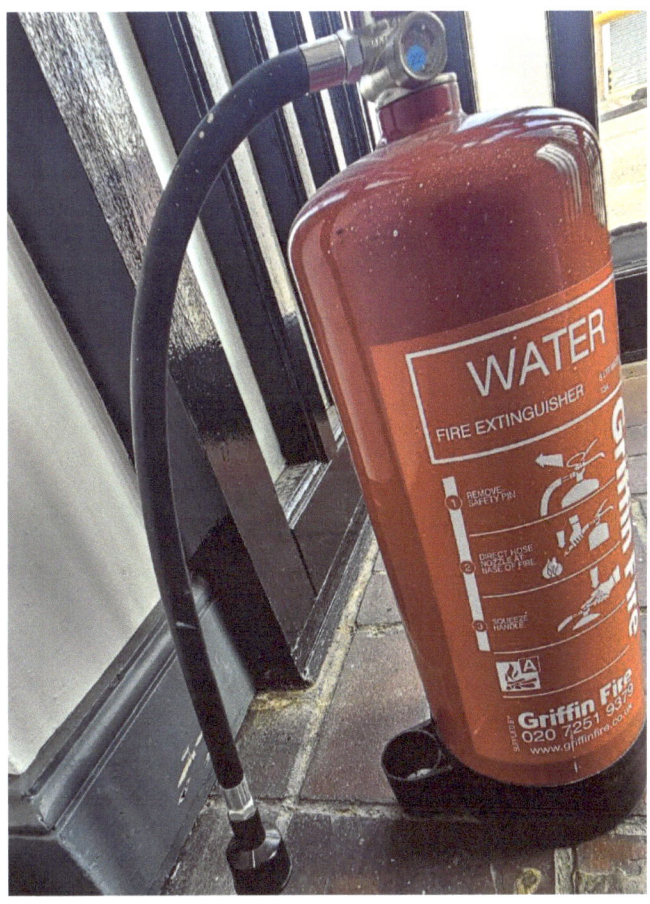

Colour	**95% red, 5%** bear the **name of the extinguisher.**
Characteristics	**The indicator needle must be green.** This means the extinguisher has the right pressure. Discharge time is between **40-50 seconds.**
Extinguishing Action	Removes the heat from the burning material.
What class of fire does it extinguish?	**Class A FIRES**- Paper, wood, and textiles.
Do not use it on	Electrical fires, fuel, metal, or chip pan fires.
Method of Use	Direct the extinguisher at the base of the fire.

CARBON DIOXIDE

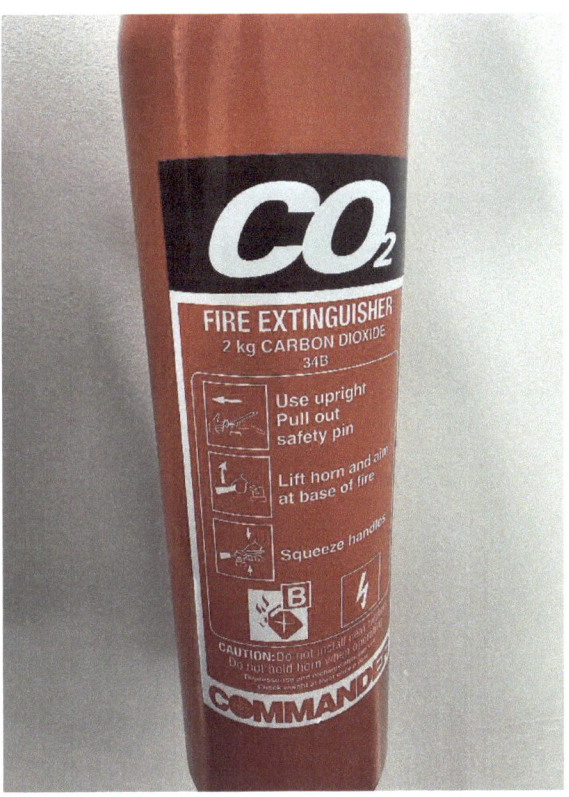

Colour	Red with a black band.
Characteristics	The intact seal should indicate it is full. Discharge time is between 20-30 seconds.
What it does	It vaporises liquid gas, which consequently displaces the oxygen around the fire.
What class of fire is it best for	- Electrical fires - Live electrical equipment - Class B fires-flammable liquids
Danger	- Don't use it on metal fires. - The gas may be harmful- evacuate the area as soon as it is used.

DRY POWDER

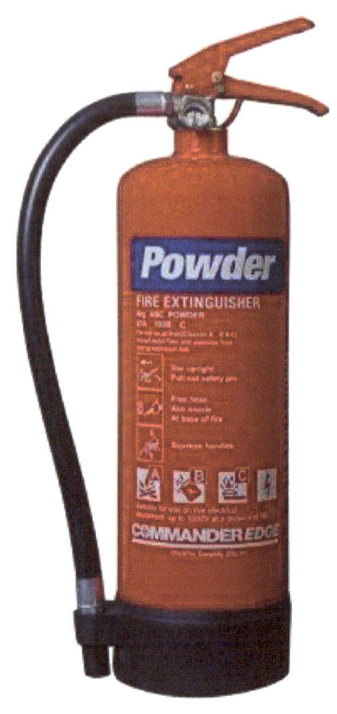

Colour	Red with blue indicator band.
Characteristics	Stored in a pressure-nitrogen cartridge. The indicator gauge needle in green. indicates the right pressure. Available in various sizes.
Extinguishing action	Drives the flame to smother and cool.
Classes of fire best for	A B C D electrical fires. Great for car engine fires.
Danger	Don't use on-chip fan fires. It can cause extensive damage to electrical fires. Create an extensive mess if used indoors. Has a limited cooling effect.
Method of use	Attack the fire by focusing the discharge nozzle at the base of the flame. Attack the flame with a rapid sweeping motion. Drive the flame to the far edge until they are out.

FOAM

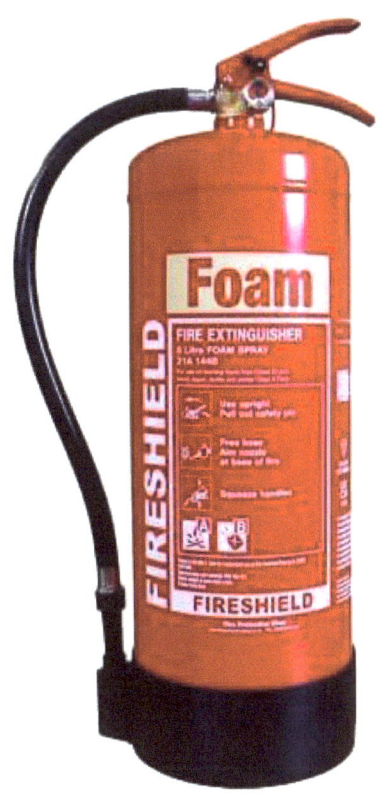

Colour	Red with cream indicator band.
Characteristic	The indicator gauge is green, indicating correct pressure. Available in varying sizes.
Action	Forms a blanket of foam over the surface of the burning liquid.
Best for	Class B fires.
Danger	Don't use it on live electrical equipment. Don't use it on chips/fat pans or metal fires. Avoid contact with eyes as it is an irritant.
Method of use	Spray above the liquid so the foam can build and flow across it.

LITHIUM EX FIRE EXTINGUISHER

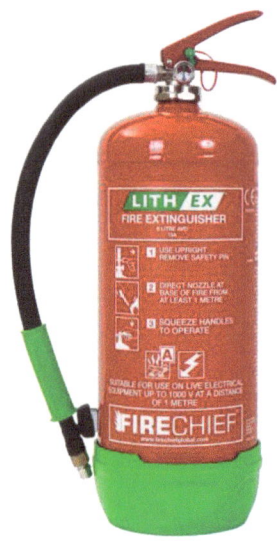

The Lithium EX is a new fire extinguisher, which is Designed to be used on fires Involving lithium batteries. This is the only extinguisher on the market, that can be used on lithium battery Fires. They can also be used on class A and electrical fires. This extinguisher works by cooling and depositing a layer of platelets, which starve the fire of oxygen and prevent re-Ignition.

Colour

Red with green indicator label and green bottom.

Characteristics

Stored pressure – air excellent.

Extinguishing action

Lith-Ex extinguishers contain Aqueous Vermiculite Dispersion (AVD), a revolutionary fire extinguishing agent. The water content of the extinguisher cools the fire source while the Vermiculite platelets encapsulate the fuel source, creating a thermal barrier to prevent the propagation of the fire.

Best for

It can be used on class A and E type fires and live electrical equipment up to 1000V.

Method of use

The jet must be directed at the base of the flames and kept moving across the area of the fire.

WET CHEMICAL FIRE EXTINGUISHER

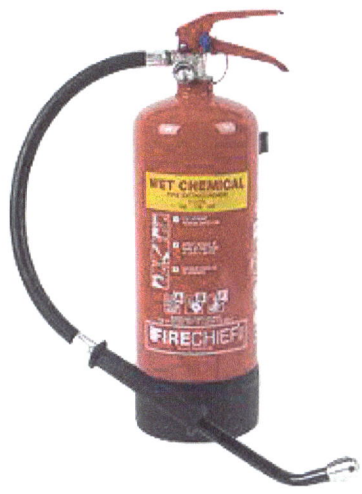

Colour- Red with a yellow band.

How it works- the chemical forms a thick foam-like blanket over the surface of the burning oil or fat, which prevents oxygen from reaching the fire and smothers the flame.

Best for: Class F fires, cooking fats, oils, and Class A fires.

Not suitable for: live electrical equipment.

How to use it: slowly squeeze the lever to discharge the wet chemical, spraying it in slow circular motions.

WATER MIST (DRY WATER MIST) FIRE EXTINGUISHER

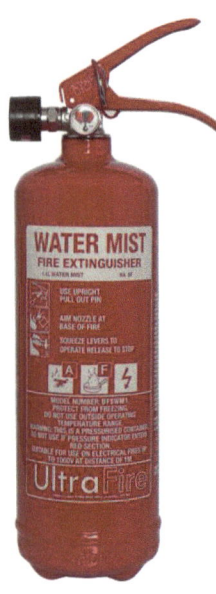

- These are designed to discharge water droplets.

- The nozzle is designed to create microscopic mist, which reduces the oxygen content around the fire.

- Creates a cooling blanket over the heat and prevents re-ignition.

- **Why they are suitable for electrical equipment/fire:**

➢ They have passed the 35KV di-electrical test (a test for the electrical safety of water-based fire extinguishers).

➢ Contain de-ionised water, which makes them suitable for fighting electrical fires from a minimum distance of 1 m.

➢ Non-harmful and non-poisonous to humans and furniture.

➢ Suitable for Class A, B, C, and F fires and electrical equipment up to 1000v.

➢ 1005 environmentally friendly.

Method of use:

The jet must be directed at the base of the flames and kept moving across the area of the fire. Any hot spots should be sought out after the main fire is extinguished.

Fire Hose

Characteristics:

Approximately 30 metres long.

Pre-set controls should mean that it is charged with

water and ready for use.

Usually, wall-mounted in or out of a container and labelled

Branch for jet or spray.

Extinguishing action:

Mainly by cooling the burning material.

Best for

A class fires- wood, paper, textiles.

Danger:

Do not use on live electrical equipment, fuel, metal, or chip

pan fires.

Method of use:

Used by a minimum team of 2, ideally 3, for doors and

feeding from real.

It can be very awkward when going through doors.

The jet must be aimed at the base of the flames and kept moving across the fire area. If an isolating valve is fitted, it should be opened before the hose is unreeled.

Do not get too brave with an unlimited supply of water- if the fire is too big, get out.

FIRE BLANKET

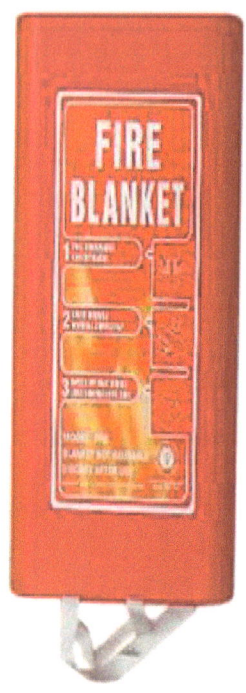

Characteristics:

Usually located in kitchens

Extinguishing action:

Smothering Best for

- ➤ Chip pan fires
- ➤ Small A class fires

Method of use:

The blanket should be placed carefully over the fire, taking care to shield the hands. Care should be taken not to wave the flames towards the user or bystanders.

Once used, it requires replacing.

- Usually located in kitchens.
- Ideal for chip pan fires.
- Starves the fire of oxygen.
- Once used, it requires replacing.
- It can be used for human fires.

RISK ASSESSMENT

<u>Definition</u>

This is an organised look at work activities and workplaces to determine what could cause harm and then take steps to minimise or avoid them.

A business has a legal duty to minimise the risk of fire in the workplace. One way of doing this is to carry out a risk assessment. It is the responsibility of the responsible to carry out a risk assessment.

The role of the responsible person or those assisting him is to look around for risks and fire hazards, establish how to evacuate the building, review action plans, and identify the equipment needed to fight the fire and prevent fire.

Hazard- something that has the potential to cause harm.

Risk- a risk is the chance, high or low, of that harm occurring.

Preparations before a risk

Assessment

- Tour of the workplace

- A tour of the workplace is vital when done as part of your preparation for a risk assessment.

- Listen to the concerns of colleagues and staff. They are the ones on the ground. Listen to their suggestions.

- Consult others with whom you have responsibility for the premises.

For fire risk assessments, there are five steps that you need to take:

Step 1: Identify potential fire hazards in the workplace. For example, electrical fires and to deal with this by good housekeeping, testing appliances, and working properly. Maintain electrical systems.

Step 2: Decide who (e.g., employees, visitors) might be in danger in the event of a fire, in the workplace, or while trying to escape from it, and note their location.

Step 3: Evaluate the risks arising from the hazards and decide whether your existing fire precautions are adequate or whether more should be done to get rid of the hazard or to control the risks (e.g., by improving the fire precautions).

Step 4: Record your findings and the details of the action you took as a result. Tell your employees about your findings.

Step 5: Keep the assessment under review and revise it when necessary. Make sure they are up-to-date.

Sample fire risk assessment

Risk assessment

Part 1: Background

You should aim to complete this section in 150 - 200 words.

Topic	Comments
Name of organisation*	ABCDE FOODS
Site location*	A3-A4 EVERSHED INDUSTRIAL ESTATE, BETWEEN ROAD, LONDON N40 0DY
Number of workers	50
General description of the organisation	ABCDE FOODS is a produce supplier based in North London. They source, import, package, distribute, supply, and market over 200 lines of fresh fruits and vegetables to the wholesale and retail trades. They sell citrus fruits, tropical fruits, and Mediterranean selections such as figs, pomegranates, and watermelon. It is headquartered in North London but has branches in South London and Manchester. It also has additional facilities in Holland and Spain. They do over 500 deliveries a week, covering the whole of London, and the vast majority of their work is carried out from their North London branch.
Description of the area to be included in the risk assessment	The
Any other relevant information	

* If you're worried about confidentiality, you can invent a false name and location for your organisation, but all other information provided must be factual.

You should aim to complete this section in 100 - 200 words.
Note: This section can be completed after you have completed your risk assessment.

Outline how the risk assessment was carried out. This should include: • sources of information consulted; • who you spoke to and • How you identified: - the hazards; - what is already being done, and - any additional controls/actions that may be required.	I started the risk assessment by researching information on the website of the HSE relating to risk assessment for warehouses and offices. I prepared a checklist of hazards and risks to look out for. I spoke to the operational office, which also acts as the company's health and safety manager. I asked the employees to describe the dangers of the jobs they carry out and elicited suggestions on how accidents and illnesses can be prevented. Evidence of the trends of accidents by seeking permission from the health and safety manager to see the accident report books covering the last 3 years. I walked around the warehouse and the office, which was adjacent to the warehouse, and looked at hazards that could reasonably be expected to cause harm. I was informed that there was a serious incident about a year ago when a forklift reversed and injured a staff member during the night shift. I also noticed that the office had multiple extension sockets, which posed a fire risk. Electrical safety and you- a brief guide Health and safety at work, 1974 Workplace (health, safety, and welfare) regulation Maintaining portable electrical equipment Warehouse and storage- a guide HSE: sample risk assessment 12 common warehouse hazards-seton What does a slip and trip accident cost? HSE

Part 2: Risk Assessment

Organisation name:
Date of assessment:
Scope of risk assessment:

Hazard category and hazard	Who might be harmed and how?	What are you already doing?	What further controls/actions are required?	Timescales for further actions to be completed (within ...)	Responsible Person's job title
FALLING FROM HEIGHTS 1. Risk of objects from heights 2. Goods falling from pallets 3. Materials falling from poorly loaded vehicles 4. Goods falling from damaged racking 5. Maintenance work involving climbing heights	The warehouse staff, forklift operators, customers on the premises to inspect produce they want to buy, cleaners, and contractors could die or suffer from serious injuries if objects fall on them. Maintenance staff could die or suffer serious injuries when fixing bulbs or lighting.	• We currently arrange periodic inspections of stepladders and ladders for faulty legs, rails, platforms, joints, and hinges. The inspections also check the wheels and brakes to ensure they are not faulty. • Warehouse staff are trained in the safe operation of the racking system. • Our company policy forbids climbing on racking. Any warehouse staff seen leaving platforms and climbing on racking will face the company's disciplinary procedure. • We also use renewable guards to minimise the risk of damage from accidental impact. All corner uprights	Current safety measures are sufficient. No further action is needed. Signs are missing on some racking systems. This must be replaced. There is a need for continued reinforcement of this information through emails. No further action is needed.	1 month 2 weeks 1 month	Warehouse manager Maintenance Supervisor Warehouse Manager

Hazard category and hazard	Who might be harmed and how?	What are you already doing?	What further controls/actions are required?	Timescales for further actions to be completed (within …)	Responsible Person's job title
		are provided with protective devices in conspicuous colours.	No further action is needed.		
		• Maintenance of our lighting and the changing of bulbs are carried out.	There is a need to take a look at the last two reports.		
		• Our racking is regularly inspected by the person responsible for racking safety (PRRS).	No further action is necessary.		
		• The loading bay is restricted to staff working in the area.			
MANUAL HANDLING **1. Musculoskeletal Disorders** such as lower back pain, neck pain, and upper limb disorders due to: a. Heavy lifting, repetitive order picking b. Bending and twisting c. Exerting too much force	Agency workers, warehouse staff, forklift operators, and contractors may suffer from lower back pain, neck pain, and upper limb disorders. These musculoskeletal injuries can be caused by heavy lifting, repetitive order picking,	• The company takes the risks of musculoskeletal injuries seriously. Manual handling tasks are inevitable in the warehouse. Bearing that in mind, we ensure that any risk from manual handling is minimised. We invest in mechanical handling devices such as pallet trucks, trolleys, and scissor lifts.	No further action is necessary. No further action is necessary.		

27

Hazard category and hazard	Who might be harmed and how?	What are you already doing?	What further controls/actions are required?	Timescales for further actions to be completed (within …)	Responsible Person's job title
d. Working too long without breaks 2. Pulling and pushing roll cages	bending and twisting, repeating an action frequently, prolonged working in an uncomfortable position, exerting too much force, and working too long without breaks. A warehouse staff pulling and pushing a roll cage that is overloaded or moving 3 to 5 empty, nested roll cages at one time and not following the correct lifting methods for loading and unloading the roll cage is at risk of suffering from musculoskeletal injuries.	• We provide regular manual handling training to our staff. Staff are trained not to overload roll cages or move more than 3 or 5 empty cages simultaneously. • All our roll cages are regularly inspected and maintained. We look for faulty wheels and encourage warehouse staff to report any protruding sharp edges on roll cages. • Staff are trained on the right way to lift to avoid lower back or upper limb disorders. • Staff are encouraged to take their breaks to avoid working too long without breaks.	No further action is needed. Remind staff through emails to update knowledge on our online manual handling course. No further action is necessary.	1 month	Health and Safety Manager

Hazard category and hazard	Who might be harmed and how?	What are you already doing?	What further controls/actions are required?	Timescales for further actions to be completed (within ...)	Responsible Person's job title
LOAD HANDLING EQUIPMENT 1. Forklift truck Crashing into other vehicles, visitors, and staff 2. Objects from forklift trucks	Forklift operators, warehouse staff, members of the public visiting the warehouse, visiting drivers, contractors, and cleaners. The risk that any of them could be struck by lift trucks, Lift trucks cause injuries through collisions with other vehicles on the premises and other objects. Objects falling from the forklift and injuring visiting drivers, customers, or warehouse staff. Forklift operator falling out of the forklift. The forklift tips over. Staff may be crushed by the mast.	The warehouse uses a counterbalanced forklift truck and is inspected and examined regularly as required by LOLER and PUMER. Members of the public are not allowed into forklift operating areas, and where such visits are allowed, we insist on the wearing of the appropriate PPE- high visibility jackets/coats and the right protective footwear, but unfortunately, we still sometimes encounter staff who do not wear the right PPE on the warehouse floor. Employees have restricted access to lift truck operating areas, and our forklifts have flashing beacons.	No further action is necessary. We have noticed lapses here. There have been reports that this is not being enforced rigorously. Line managers must highlight this through toolbox talk. No further action is necessary.	1 month	Warehouse Manager
3. Accidents involving roll cages	Customers on the warehouse floor, visiting drivers, cleaners, and forklift drivers	We maintain a rigorous inspection and maintenance regime.	No further action is necessary.		

Hazard category and hazard	Who might be harmed and how?	What are you already doing?	What further controls/actions are required?	Timescales for further actions to be completed (within …)	Responsible Person's job title
	can be injured when roll cages controlled by warehouse staff collide with them due to jammed or faulty wheels or protruding sharp edges resulting from a lack of proper monitoring.				
ELECTRICAL SAFETY Multiple Cables/leads are connected to the floor cleaner in the warehouse c. battery charging equipment	Contractors, warehouse staff, visiting drivers, cleaning staff, and other visitors to the premises can die, suffer from burns, or suffer from electric shock from damage to the plug, lead, fraying, cuts, or heavy scuffing. Especially at risk from damaged cables are cleaners, warehouse staff, and visitors to the warehouse if the cables/lead connected to	We carry out PAT testing annually on all portable electrical equipment. All fixed installations are maintained and inspected regularly. All our earthed (class 1) floor cleaners undergo a visual inspection every 6-12 months and a combined inspection and testing every 1-2 years. Our cables/leads plugs connected to floor cleaners, mains voltage extension leads, and battery charging equipment undergo a formal visual inspection	There is no record of any PAT tests done in the past 12 months. There are no records of any inspections or maintenance done in the last 12 months. Check when the last inspection was done and when the next one is due. No record of any inspection in the last 14 months.	1 month 1 month 1 month 1 month	**Warehouse Manager/Health and Safety Manager** **Warehouse Manager** **Maintenance Supervisor** **Health and Safety Manager**

Hazard category and hazard	Who might be harmed and how?	What are you already doing?	What further controls/actions are required?	Timescales for further actions to be completed (within ...)	Responsible Person's job title
	floor cleaners are damaged. A forklift operator can die or suffer serious injury if they touch the terminals when they are connected or if the current is passing through them. The forklift battery charger can cause an electric shock due to the wrong terminal connection and touching the wire incorrectly.	every 6 months-4 years.			
FIRE SAFETY 1. Storage of combustible materials at the entrance of the warehouse 2. Arson 3. Blockage of fire escape routes with loaded pallets 4. Ignition by faulty electrical equipment	Visitors to the warehouse, members of the public, visiting drivers, and customers can get injured or die as a result of combustible materials meeting an ignition source. Smoking cigarettes and encountering empty cardboard boxes.	There are sufficient storage containers for combustible materials. Combustible materials are not allowed to accumulate on the warehouse floor or any other part of the site. Storage areas are properly monitored. We operate a strictly no-smoking policy. We carry out regular fire drills.	Have more fire marshals. Instruct staff to report any faults immediately. Remove the waste skip from the front of the warehouse.	1 month 1 month 1 month	Health and Safety Manager Warehouse Manager Warehouse Manager

Hazard category and hazard	Who might be harmed and how?	What are you already doing?	What further controls/actions are required?	Timescales for further actions to be completed (within …)	Responsible Person's job title
	The position of the waste storage container in front of the warehouse can be a lure to arsonists. Also, warehouse staff, customers visiting the business, contractors, and other staff members can be injured or die from fire if pallets and other obstructions to the fire exit routes continue. Also, faulty electrical equipment can be particularly harmful to visiting drivers, customers, cleaners, warehouse staff, and forklift drivers due to electric shock.	Fire escape routes and fire doors are clearly marked with regular signs. The building has been designed using fire-retardant materials. Our fire safety contractors regularly test our fire testing and service our fire extinguishers. Fire training is provided to our staff on the use of fire extinguishers. There are fire detection systems and fire alarms in place. Staff are aware to keep all fire escape routes clear of obstructions.			
SLIPS, TRIPS, AND FALL 1. Obstructions on the warehouse floor by articles and substances	Cleaners, contractors, warehouse staff, visiting drivers, customers, and visiting members of the public slip,	Our workflows are planned to ensure goods and equipment are not obstructing or projecting into places where people walk. We provide enough storage	The anti-slip floor coating in the warehouse is damaged in parts. Maintenance is required – replace	1 month	General Manager

32

Hazard category and hazard	Who might be harmed and how?	What are you already doing?	What further controls/actions are required?	Timescales for further actions to be completed (within ...)	Responsible Person's job title
2. Spillage of juice loaded on pallets and cages 3. Waste materials are allowed to accumulate on the warehouse floor	trip, and fall when waste materials such as shrink, stretch wrap, or label backing are left on the warehouse floor. This can lead to death or serious injury. Spillage of juice loaded on pallets or cages can cause injury to cleaners, warehouse staff, visiting drivers, and members of the public visiting the warehouse when they slip and fall.	for busy periods to prevent goods or other items from being stored in walkways and traffic routes. We plan waste disposal to ensure waste items do not accumulate on the warehouse floor. All materials on traffic routes are cleared without delay. We provide good lighting. And insists on staff and visitors wearing suitable footwear in the warehouse. We discourage rushing around the warehouse. Any spillage anywhere on the premises is cleaned off immediately.	damaged and worn coatings. Spillages still happen despite our best efforts. Remove contamination quickly. Spot clean spills, and dry mob large wet areas. No further action is required.	2 month	
MENTAL ILLNESS **Stress** 1. Shift work 2. Delivery targets 3. Online order delivery	Warehouse staff, delivery	Our aim is to control the workload of our staff.	This is constantly under review. Line managers are	2 months	Line Manager (warehouse)

Hazard category and hazard	Who might be harmed and how?	What are you already doing?	What further controls/actions are required?	Timescales for further actions to be completed (within …)	Responsible Person's job title
	drivers, forklift drivers, and logistic staff can develop a mental illness due to the stress resulting from working long hours. About 30% of the company staff are over 40 years old and therefore particularly vulnerable to inflexible shift work. Stress can lead to fatigue, accidents, injuries, and ill health. Unrealistic order targets can adversely affect those in the logistic team and delivery drivers if they continue to work long hours with limited rest periods.	Include employees in planning and carrying out events. Our company has a comprehensive policy on mental health. There is an emphasis on managing return from sickness absences. We discuss the format of their return well in advance of any given return date. Shift work is organised to take into account personal circumstances.	encouraged to speak to staff regularly about their workload or underload. This is done on an ongoing basis. No further action is required now.		
WORK-RELATED VIOLENCE 1. Physical attack 2. Harassment 3. Psychological	Warehouse staff, visiting drivers, our delivery drivers, our customer support team, and security officers can suffer work-related violence	The company operates a zero-tolerance policy on violence of any form. We will insist on prosecution if any staff member is assaulted by visitors, and	We have never received any reports of violence against our staff. However, the company recognises the importance of training to ensure this	2 months	Personnel Manager

Hazard category and hazard	Who might be harmed and how?	What are you already doing?	What further controls/actions are required?	Timescales for further actions to be completed (within ...)	Responsible Person's job title
	through harassment, physical and psychological attacks. The harassment might take the form of assault or sexual and racial abuse. Physical violence might take the form of beating, kicking, slapping, pushing, and biting. Workplace violence can lead to sick leave, displacement from work life, and possibly suicide.	where the violence is within, dismissal will be made where anyone is confirmed to have resorted to physical, psychological, or any form of harassment after a disciplinary hearing.

Openness, communication, and dialogue are encouraged right from the top of the organisation.

The company premises, including the warehouse, are well-lit, and lighting is maintained on a regular basis to increase visibility in all areas, including access, parking, and storage areas at night.

Surveillance cameras are in operation 24 hours a day in customer areas, and a beeper is installed at the warehouse reception area. | laudable record continues.

We have booked a mental first aid course for five of our employees, which shows we are not resting on our laurels.

No further action is required. | | |

Hazard category and hazard	Who might be harmed and how?	What are you already doing?	What further controls/actions are required?	Timescales for further actions to be completed (within ...)	Responsible Person's job title
VEHICLES IN AROUND THE WAREHOUSE **1. Visiting delivery drivers who do not speak English** **2. Vehicle collision** **3. Struck by vehicle**	Visiting drivers unable to read site rules and identifiable hazards can lead to injuries or fatalities to warehouse staff, contractors, and members of the public. Warehouse staff, visiting drivers, forklift operators, and members of the public visiting the site can collide with delivery vehicles while reversing in the parking areas. Lorry movement during shift change can lead to warehouse staff, contractors, and visiting members of the public getting struck and suffering injuries or fatalities.	The company receives deliveries from Europe and other countries. We recognise the difficulties such drivers may face on the company premises when arriving. Visiting drivers are made aware of hazards on the way when approaching our site so they can plan their journey. We illustrate site rules with pictograms to cover expected foreign languages. There are separate areas for car parking for lorry and lift truck operations. Additionally, there is increased lighting and visibility. No lorry movements during shift change. Vehicles and pedestrians have an adequate separation between them.	The foreign languages currently covered are Spanish, Dutch, and Turkish. As we are beginning to see more Polish and Romanian visiting drivers, there is a need to cover those languages as well. Exclude non-essential personnel from areas where vehicles are reversing. No further action is necessary. No further action is needed.	1 month 1 week	Operational Manager/Warehouse Manager Warehouse Manager

Hazard category and hazard	Who might be harmed and how?	What are you already doing?	What further controls/actions are required?	Timescales for further actions to be completed (within ...)	Responsible Person's job title
HAZARDOUS SUBSTANCES **1. Cleaning agents** **a. Bleach cleaning fluids** **2. Vehicle exhaust fumes discharge of carbon monoxide** **3. Forklift charging batteries** **a. Release of hydrogen and potential for an explosion** **b. Spillage of acid**	Cleaners are exposed to bleach and cleaning fluids. These chemicals can cause respiratory problems as well as an irritating effect on the skin. Delivery drivers are exposed to fumes from delivering vehicles, which can have fatal consequences if carbon monoxide is inhaled at dangerous levels. Forklift drivers, cleaners, and warehouse staff may be exposed to the dangerous effect of hydrogen gas emitted while charging forklift batteries. The acid spillage can lead to serious burns to forklift drivers, warehouse staff, and cleaners.	Cleaners undergo COSHH training, so they are familiar with chemical agents that cause skin irritation/dermatitis. They are required to wear gloves and appropriate footwear. They know that PPE is not an option; it must always be worn during work. They are trained to put up signs to warn other staff and visitors when the floor is wet or where there is spillage. The doors to the warehouse are always open to encourage ventilation, as is the loading bay. In terms of carbon monoxide poisoning due to exposure to fumes from delivery vehicles, drivers are encouraged to turn off engines once parked. In terms of the release of hydrogen when forklift batteries are being charged, this only takes place in designated and well-ventilated	• So far, there have been no complaints of cleaners suffering from skin problems relating to cleaning agents used in their work. If that comes to our attention, we will introduce alternative and safer cleaning products. No further action is required at the moment, but periodic review is encouraged.	6 months 6 months 6 months	Sarah Goodwill (Cleaning Supervisor)

Hazard category and hazard	Who might be harmed and how?	What are you already doing?	What further controls/actions are required?	Timescales for further actions to be completed (within ...)	Responsible Person's job title
		areas of the warehouse. Forklift operators are required to follow a safe system of work and are required to wear gloves and goggles. The warehouse also has an eye-wash station in case of a splash of chemicals to the eyes.	No further action is required at the moment, but periodic review is necessary to maintain standards.		
LONE WORKING 1. Threat of violence 2. Lone workers whose first language is not English	Cleaners, night shift workers, delivery drivers, maintenance and repair staff, contractors, our warehouse staff, and any staff who work by themselves without close or direct supervision are particularly vulnerable to the threat of violence. Many of our delivery drivers are of Turkish origin and, as a result, are particularly vulnerable when working on their own, as communication may be a	Our staff, especially our delivery drivers, are trained to cope with unexpected circumstances with the potential for violence and aggression. Our delivery drivers have pre-agreed intervals of regular contact with a supervisor on site. Drivers are issued with radios, and they all carry mobile phones. All delivery drivers carry a first aid kit in the vehicle. New drivers are accompanied for the first month while on the job.	The company prides itself on the procedures in place for lone working but is not complacent. We are constantly reviewing our lone working procedures and providing online training to our staff. Now, no further action is necessary.	6 months 6 months	Operational Manager Health and Safety Manager

Hazard category and hazard	Who might be harmed and how?	What are you already doing?	What further controls/actions are required?	Timescales for further actions to be completed (within …)	Responsible Person's job title
	problem for some of them.				

Part 3: Prioritise 3 actions with justification for the selection.

Suggested word counts
Moral and financial arguments for all actions: 300 to 350 words
For EACH action:
Specific legal arguments: 100 to 150 words
Likelihood AND severity: 75 to 150 words
How effective the action is likely to be in controlling the risk: 100 to 150 words

Moral and financial arguments for ALL actions

Moral, general legal, and financial arguments	**FIRE SAFETY: Arrange to remove the skip from the front of the warehouse.** The moral, legal, and financial arguments for this action have been explained in the justification for Action 1 **ELECTRICAL SAFETY: Inspection and examination of portable electrical equipment and battery charging equipment.** The moral, legal, and financial arguments have been explained in the justification for Action 2 **SLIP, TRIP, AND FALL- The anti-slip floor coating in the warehouse is damaged in parts. Maintenance required – replace damaged and worn coatings.** The moral, legal, and financial arguments have been explained in the justification for Action 3

Justification for Action 1

Action	The action I am prioritising is fire safety. 1. **Arrange to remove the skip from the front of the warehouse.** **Moral argument** Our company is morally obligated to protect all employees and visitors to our premises. Employees are the most valuable asset to a company. The skip outside for storing waste is a fire hazard. Though the company has a no-smoking policy, this policy does not stop an accidental fire from occurring if a visitor ignites the combustible materials in the skip with a smoking cigarette. Staff working inside the warehouse might be trapped inside, which can lead to serious injuries or fatalities. It is morally indefensible for our staff to come to work and end up being injured or killed over an issue that could have been easily dealt with. If they are injured, there will be pain and suffering for them personally and for those members of their families that have to help them recover. We make profits from the efforts put in daily by our staff. Our duty to provide income to our staff also extends to our moral responsibility to ensure their safety. **LEGAL ARGUMENT** The employer has a general duty to ensure the health, safety, and welfare of employees so far as is reasonably practicable and to ensure the workplace is safe. (Health and Safety at Work Act 1974-s2). We also have specific duties under the "Regulatory Reform (Fire Safety) Order 2005". Our company is obliged to take such general fire precautions as will ensure, so far as is reasonably practicable, the safety of any of its employees and non-employees who might be on the premises. Leaving a skip with combustible materials

in front of a warehouse poses a fire risk to our employees as well as visitors to the premises.

Implementing the action as recommended satisfies the requirement of the law to carry out a suitable and sufficient fire risk assessment.

Failure to comply with the regulation can lead to enforcement action by the Health and Safety Executive. The HSE has the power to investigate a material breach of any health and safety legislation, and if they conclude that such a material breach is serious enough and must be remedied, they will write to us to take action to deal with the material breach. If the notification is necessary, this will usually be sent after a visit by an inspector, and our company will be liable to pay the fees for their investigation, which is usually £157 per hour. It is unlikely that having a skip full of combustible material might lead to prosecution. Still, if someone were to die due to the ignition of the materials in the skip, a prosecution might ensue if it is shown that management was aware of the fire risk posed by the skip in front of the warehouse.

FINANCIAL ARGUMENT

The financial impact of fire on our organisation can be devastating. Our company will incur massive expenses rebuilding the warehouse, and our products will be damaged and must be replaced. Additionally, while we are rebuilding, there will inevitably be lost production time; if there are casualties, there is the cost of compensating relatives. Individual employees injured as a result of the fire will sue the company for personal injury and loss of income. Even if some of the financial impacts will be borne by our insurance company, the overall cost of premiums on our insurance will skyrocket and dent our profit margin.

I estimate that the cost of relocating and rebuilding more durable storage containers for our combustible wastes will be no more than £10,000-£15,000. In contrast, the financial cost of inaction will be £5 million in the event of fatality, injury, or both.

Specific legal arguments	**LEGAL ARGUMENTS** **REGULATORY REFORM (FIRE SAFETY) REGULATION 2005** The employer has a general duty to ensure the health, safety, and welfare of employees so far as is reasonably practicable and to ensure the workplace is safe. **HEALTH AND SAFETY AT WORK ACT 1974-S2.** We also have specific duties under the **Regulatory Reform (Fire Safety) Order of 2005.** Our company is required to take such general fire precautions as will ensure, so far as is reasonably practicable, the safety of any of its employees as well as non-employees who might be on the premises. Leaving a skip with combustible materials in front of a warehouse poses a fire risk to our employees as well as visitors to the premises. Implementing the action as recommended satisfies the requirement of the law to carry out a suitable and sufficient fire risk assessment. Failure to implement the action will be a material breach of the requirement of **MANAGING OF HEALTH AND SAFETY AT WORK REGULATION 1999** Our company is also in breach of **Section 2(1)(2) of the Health and Safety at Work Act 1974.** We owe our employees a duty, as far as is reasonably practicable, to ensure their health, safety, and welfare, and a specific duty in s2 to ensure a safe working environment. The material breach of the law stated above could lead to enforcement action by the health and safety inspectors of the HSE.

	ENFORCEMENT ACTION The actions listed above are so serious that we could face enforcement actions from the HSE inspectors if they are of the view that there has been a material breach. A material breach that leads to a notification to correct the breach of the law will incur a fee for their investigation, which is £157 per hour. If the breach of law is not corrected or leads to death or serious injuries, our company or even the directors of the company can face prosecution. **The Company's Directors Disqualification Act 1986** can lead to our directors being disqualified from holding the office of directors in the future. There is the additional risk that individuals within the company could face prosecution for **gross negligence and manslaughter.** And our company was charged with **corporate manslaughter** if any staff members were to die from injuries sustained from the breach of duty.
Consideration of likelihood AND severity	Should we fail to act, I will assess the likelihood of uncontrolled fire as medium to high. Our business is located near a large council estate. Due to the COVID-19 lockdown, the youths who live in the estate have a lot of time on their hands, and our CCTV cameras have seen several of them straying into the business park where our business is located. A large fire can lead to serious injuries. According to the home office, there were 231 fire-related fatalities in England at the end of June 2020. According to the Chief Fire Officer's Association, 60% of businesses affected by fire never recover.
How effective the action is likely to be in controlling the risk. This should include: • the intended impact of the action; • justification for the timescale that you indicated in your risk assessment and • whether you think the action will fully control the risk.	All combustible wastes are deposited into the waste storage outside the warehouse. Relocating it to the back of the warehouse ensures it is no longer accessible to intruders and arsonists. While the risk of fire will not be eliminated, at the very least, we are reducing the risk by relocating the storage to the back of the warehouse. In the event of a major fire, our staff will not be trapped inside the warehouse. They will have the front of the warehouse as an escape route. **JUSTIFICATION FOR THE TIMESCALE** The risk will be reviewed within a month of the work being completed, and subsequently, the risk assessment will be reviewed every six months. I reckon that because of COVID-19, due to the drop in business in all sectors of the economy, any contractor recruited will be quite happy to complete the work within the set timescale. **WILL THE ACTION FULLY CONTROL THE RISK?** No control measure put in place will prevent fire 100%. There is always a residual risk of fire, especially arson. But with the CCTV and the containers constructed with fire-retardant materials there, I am optimistic that the measures proposed will be highly effective.

Justification for Action 2

Action	
	ELECTRICAL SAFETY: Inspection and examination of portable electrical equipment and battery charging equipment.

The action I am prioritising is the hazard-due inspection and examination of electrical equipment and battery charging equipment in the warehouse.

MORAL - Though the health and safety officer claims there is a regular regime of testing and examination of portable and electrical equipment and the forklift battery charger, there does not appear to be a record to back this up. This inconsistency is morally indefensible, as we are talking about people's lives. If there is regular testing and examination of this workplace equipment, then our records should show this. The forklift battery charger can cause exposure to acid, which can damage the skin and clothes of our employees. It can burn skin and clothes. Hydrogen gas emitted during charging can cause an explosion. Also, electric shock can occur due to the wrong terminal connection or by touching the wires. Burns, electric shock, and injuries due to fire can lead to life-changing injuries. Our employees do not deserve any injuries while working for us. We also have to think about the family that must care for them and the psychological impact of post-traumatic stress caused by these experiences.

LEGAL:

Electricity at Work Regulation 1989

Our company must ensure that, as far as reasonably practicable, all electrical equipment, including portable electrical equipment and installations, is maintained to prevent danger. This is the requirement of the Electricity at Work Regulation of 1989. The fact that we are unable to show proof of any recent maintenance and inspection of our electrical equipment means we are not able to show evidence of risk assessment, which is a legal requirement. We are also in breach of the Health and Safety at Work Act, Section 2, which requires us to ensure that the workplace is safe and that we are ensuring the health and safety of our employees at work.

The actions listed above are so serious that we could face enforcement actions from the HSE inspectors if they are of the view that there has been a material breach. A material breach that is so serious can lead to a notification to correct the breach of the law. They charge a fee for their investigation, which is £157 per hour. If the breach of law is not corrected or leads to death or serious injuries, our company or even the directors of the company can face prosecution.

FINANCIAL

The actions highlighted are those that can lead to serious injuries and possibly death, especially from electric shock. A Hydrogen explosion can lead to fire, which can affect the operation of the business. The business will have to close. Even though such losses are insurable, prosecution by the HSE inspectors is

	uninsurable. According to the Chief Fire Officer's Association, 60% of businesses that have been affected by fire do not recover.

Our employees and their families will be seeking compensation for injuries sustained or from death arising from any injuries.

Our company will be liable for sick pay, medical costs, replacement labour, and the loss of experienced staff members.

If we are found guilty of material breach, the fines imposed by HSE (HEALTH AND SAFETY EXECUTIVE) would be in the region of £1-4 million. |
| Specific legal arguments | **LEGAL ARGUMENTS**

ELECTRICITY AT WORK REGULATION 1989

Our company must ensure that, as far as reasonably practicable, all electrical equipment, including portable electrical equipment and installations, is maintained to prevent danger. This is a requirement of the Electricity at Work Regulation of 1989. The fact that we are unable to show proof of any recent maintenance and inspection of our electrical equipment means we are not able to show evidence of risk assessment, which is a legal requirement. This is a breach of the requirement of **THE MANAGING OF HEALTH AND SAFETY AT WORK REGULATION 1999.**

Our company is also in breach of **Section 2(1)(2) of the Health and Safety at Work Act 1974.** We owe our employees a duty to, as far as is reasonably practicable, ensure their health, safety, and welfare, and the specific duty in s2 is to ensure a safe working environment. The material breach of the law stated above could lead to enforcement action by the health and safety inspectors of the HSE.

ENFORCEMENT ACTION

The actions listed above are so serious that we could face enforcement actions from the HSE inspectors if they are of the view that there has been a material breach. A material breach that leads to a notification to correct the breach of the law will incur a fee for their investigation, which is £157 per hour. If the breach of law is not corrected or leads to death or serious injuries, our company or even the directors of the company can face prosecution.

The Company's Directors Disqualification Act 1986 can lead to our directors being disqualified from holding the office of directors in the future.

There is the additional risk that individuals within the company could face prosecution for **gross negligence and manslaughter.** And our company was charged with **corporate manslaughter** if any staff members were to die from injuries sustained from the breach of duty. |
| Consideration of likelihood AND severity | **LIKELIHOOD**

The failures that have been highlighted are quite serious, and the likelihood of electric shock, burns, and fire is too high if no inspection or examination has been done on portable electric equipment and the forklift battery charger for the |

	last 14 months. While records of any inspection are unavailable, it is suggested that an immediate visual examination of all portable electrical equipment and the battery charger be carried out. **SEVERITY AND CONSEQUENCES** A faulty battery charger can lead to the spillage of acid and the discharge of hydrogen, which can cause an explosion and, consequently, injuries and burns. Damaged portable electrical equipment can lead to electric shock and, consequently, the death of our employees. Our building is at risk from fire, and our staff is at risk of death, injury, or both.
How effective the action is likely to be in controlling the risk. This should include: - the intended impact of the action; - justification for the timescale that you indicated in your risk assessment and - whether you think the action will fully control the risk.	**CONTROLLING THE RISK** An immediate check of all the portable electrical equipment for faults Sockets should be positioned close to the work point so the cleaner does not have to use long leads/cables. Apart from controlling the risk of electric shock, we will be minimising the risk of trips. There ought to be a better record-keeping system for inspections and examinations carried out. **SEVERITY** **TIMESCALE** **WILL THE ACTION FULLY CONTROL THE RISK?**

Justification for Action 3

Action	**SLIP, TRIP, AND FALL-** The anti-slip floor coating in the warehouse is damaged in parts. Maintenance required – replace damaged and worn coatings. **MORAL** – On a human level, we owe a moral duty to take care of each other. No one deserves to go to work to die or get injured. Society will no doubt frown on our company's dereliction of duty, which allowed any fatality or injury to our staff. Not implementing the action could cause injury or death. Our moral duty is not just for the pain and suffering that we cause the employee but also for the stress that it causes the families of our staff who have to take care of them. We must also think of the impact that such pain will have on other members of staff who will have to deal with them or subsequently work with them if they ever recover from the injury. Society respects good standards of health and safety. According to the HSE, the cost of slip trip and fall to society is about $800 million annually. This is morally indefensible. **FINANCIAL ARGUMENT** According to HSE, the cost to employers of slips, trips, and falls in the UK is £500 million per year. **("What do slip and trip accidents cost?")**. **Our company will be impacted financially** by an increase in our company's insurance premium, as injuries and fatalities at work form part of our insurable costs. There will inevitably be delays to our production, the cost of overtime and training temporary labour will increase, not to mention the time allocated to investigation, which could be better spent on other, more productive work. The imposition of fines for investigation by HSE INSPECTORS WILL BE UNAVOIDABLE AS A CONSEQUENCE OF THEIR INVOLVEMENT. In this dynamic age of 24-hour media, the damage to our image may be irreparable. I estimate it will cost our company approximately £5,000– £7,000 to fix the damage to the floor.
Specific legal arguments	**LEGAL ARGUMENTS** **THE WORKPLACE (HEALTH AND SAFETY AND WELFARE) REGULATIONS 1992** **Regulation 12:** Every floor in a workroom shall be of suitable construction, shall have no hole, or shall be uneven or slippery. According to the regulation, workplace floors must not be uneven or slippery to the extent that they could cause someone to slip, trip, or fall; floors should be kept from obstructions, articles, and substances that could cause someone to slip, trip, or fall. Our company is in breach of Regulation 12 if the anti-slip coating on the floor remains damaged because it poses a risk of someone slipping and falling. Apart from the material breach of Regulation 12 of the 1992 Regulation, our company is also in breach of **Section 2(1)(2) of the Health and Safety at Work Act 1974.**

	We owe our employees a duty to, as far as is reasonably practicable, ensure their health, safety, and welfare, and a specific duty in s2 to ensure a safe working environment. The material breach of the law stated above could lead to enforcement action by the health and safety inspectors of the HSE. **ENFORCEMENT ACTION** The actions listed above are so serious that we could face enforcement actions from the HSE inspectors if they are of the view that there has been a material breach. A material breach that leads to a notification to correct the breach of the law will incur a fee for their investigation, which is £157 per hour. If the breach of law is not corrected or leads to death or serious injuries, our company or even the directors of the company can face prosecution. **The Company's Directors Disqualification Act 1986** can lead to our directors being disqualified from holding the office of directors in the future. There is the additional risk that individuals within the company could face prosecution for **gross negligence and manslaughter.** And our company was charged with **corporate manslaughter** if any staff members were to die from injuries sustained from the breach of duty.
Consideration of likelihood AND severity	**LIKELIHOOD** The likelihood of injury from slips, trips, and falls in a warehouse environment is high due to the various hazards in the warehouse. Our core business is importing and exporting fruits and drinks. It is clear that the risk of slips and trips cannot be fully eliminated, making it more urgent that we implement the control measures suggested in this risk assessment. SEVERITY Spillage from broken drink bottles and fruits dropped in the warehouse from damaged cartons will happen, and there will always be risks of our staff and visitors slipping and tripping on waste from unwrapped packages, empty cartons, etc. There is an even higher risk of injuries such as fractures, dislocations, and spinal and skull fractures being sustained by staff.
How effective the action is likely to be in controlling the risk. This should include: • the intended impact of the action; • justification for the timescale	**CONTROLLING THE RISK** Research by the HSE has shown that anti-slip walkways reduce slip risks in a food factory (Health and Safety Food Laboratory). **"Anti-slip walkways reduce slip risks in a large food factory.** Our company has invested in anti-slip floors, but their effect on reducing slip is eliminated if they are damaged. While installing anti-slip floors will not eliminate the risk of slipping, they will minimise the risk to a significant degree. Repairing the damaged anti-slip floor is much more cost-effective than replacing the entire anti-slip floor currently in place. **TIMESCALE** One month is sufficient time to carry out the remedial work. A longer period exposes our staff to a greater risk, and a shorter period may not be feasible because of the current government lockdown.

that you indicated in your risk assessment and • whether you think the action will fully control the risk.	**WILL THE ACTION FULLY CONTROL THE RISK?** As indicated above, repairing the damaged anti-slip floor will not totally eliminate the risk, but research has shown that having an anti-slip floor, especially an undamaged one, will not be effective in reducing the risk of slip and fall.

Part 4: Review, communicate, and check

Suggested word counts for each section:
- Planned review date or period and reasoning for this: **50 - 100 words**
- How the risk assessment findings will be communicated and who needs to know the information: **100 - 150 words**
- Follow up on the risk assessment: **100 - 150 words.**

Planned review date/period with **reasoning**	The review date for this risk assessment will be after the actions recommended have been completed, after which the risk assessment should be reviewed every 6 months. There is no need to carry out a risk assessment where no control measures suggested have been implemented.
How the risk assessment findings will be communicated **AND** who you need to tell	There are several ways that the risk assessment can be communicated, including toolbox talk with the staff, memos, emails, posting the information on noticeboards, and through a poster. However, my preferred methods of communicating the information are face-to-face meetings at the safety committee meetings, where responsible managers and safety representatives can be briefed in order for the information to be passed down to the staff. Also, through emails and posting the risk assessment on the noticeboard for staff to read.
How will you follow up on the risk assessment to check that the actions have been carried out	I will follow up on the risk assessment and ensure that the actions have been carried out by making notes of the relevant dates in my diary. I will contact the maintenance supervisor, the warehouse manager, the health and safety manager, and the general manager at the very least a week before the relevant review date to check up on progress. Once the various works have been completed, I will carry out a safety tour with the responsible manager and supervisors to ensure all of the work has been done to the required standard.

ROLE OF THE FIRE WARDEN

Fire Warden

Under the Regulatory Fire Reform Order, there must be a designated person known as the fire warden. His main role is to assist the responsible person in ensuring the building is as safe as possible from any fire risk. He has the highest responsibility.

Fire Marshal

This is someone who will assist the fire warden in executing their duties because, in the event of a fire, the fire warden cannot be everywhere simultaneously. There will be different fire marshals in different parts of the building or workplace. Assists the fire ward in the event of a fire.

The fire warden's role is not limited to when there is a fire. His responsibilities extend to the following:

- Check daily that the fire doors are not propped open and that the doors are working properly.
- Make sure the fire escape routes are clear.
- Ensure the alarm system works.
- Work with the responsible person to ensure the evacuation plans work correctly.
- Schedule fire drills and test evacuations.
- Make sure fire extinguishers are OK, in the right position, they have not been tampered with, and are clean.
- Review fire policies.
- Check for fire hazards and put preventive measures in place.
- Ensure fire Marshals are getting the right training; they know what to do in the event of an evacuation.
- Fire briefing, especially for new staff.
- Your role is really educational.

ROLE OF THE FIRE MARSHAL

- Assists the fire, Warden.
- Ensure everyone has left the building following the right route.
- Ensure those with disabilities are assisted.

- Ensure people are not carrying their bags with them.

- Ensure the doors and windows are closed.

- If there is anything within the building that you must report, then report to the fire warden when he arrives.

- Assist in the evacuation of the building.

- Fight fire if it is safe to do so.

- Move everyone to the assembly point.

- Carry out a roll call.

- Take the advice of the fire warden and the company or fire service.

- Wear the high-vis jacket in the fire kit.

FINAL SWEEP

- Plan your sweep so that you move towards the fire exit.

- Carry out a quick sweep of your area.

- If possible, turn off equipment and close doors/windows as you pass.

- Check offices, toilets, refuges (if installed), and meeting rooms.

Carry out a Roll call

- At the assembly point.

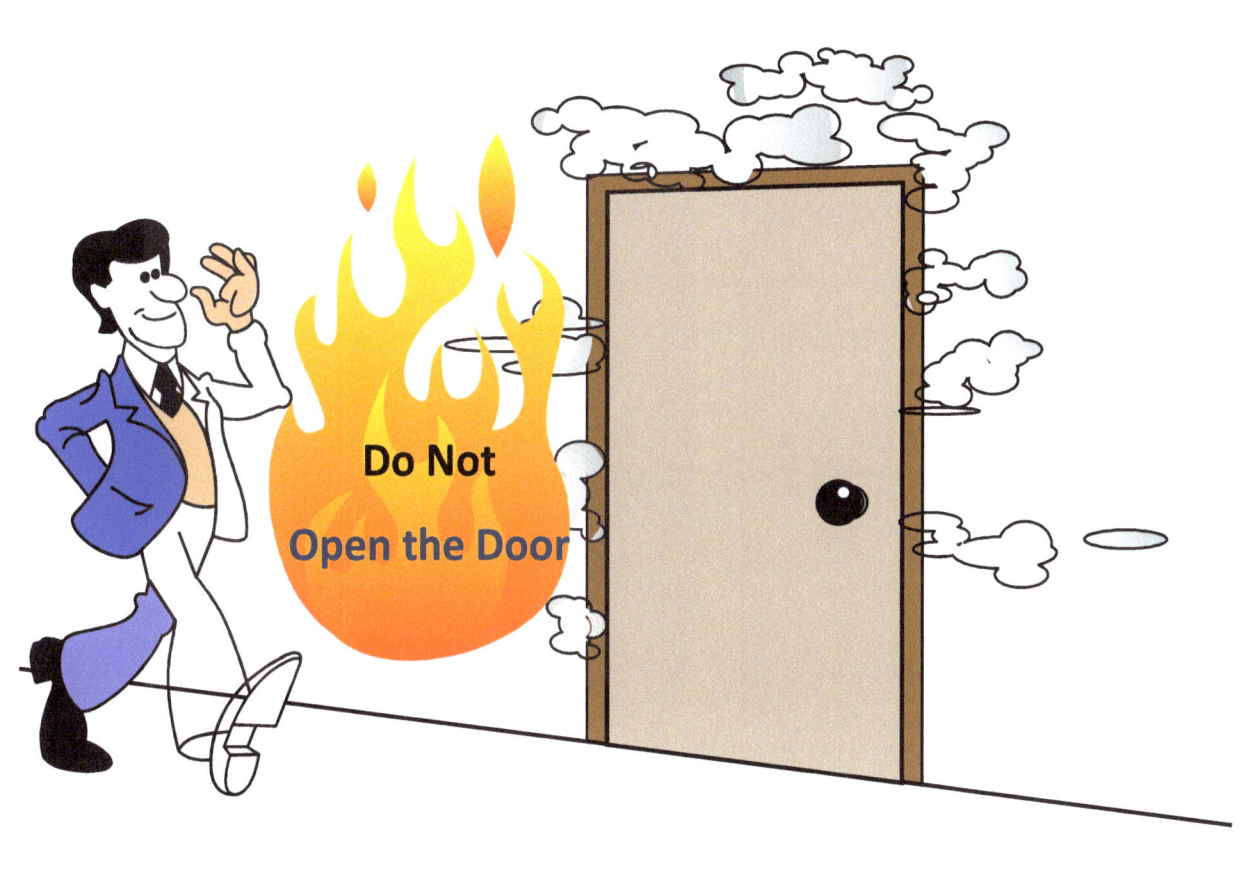
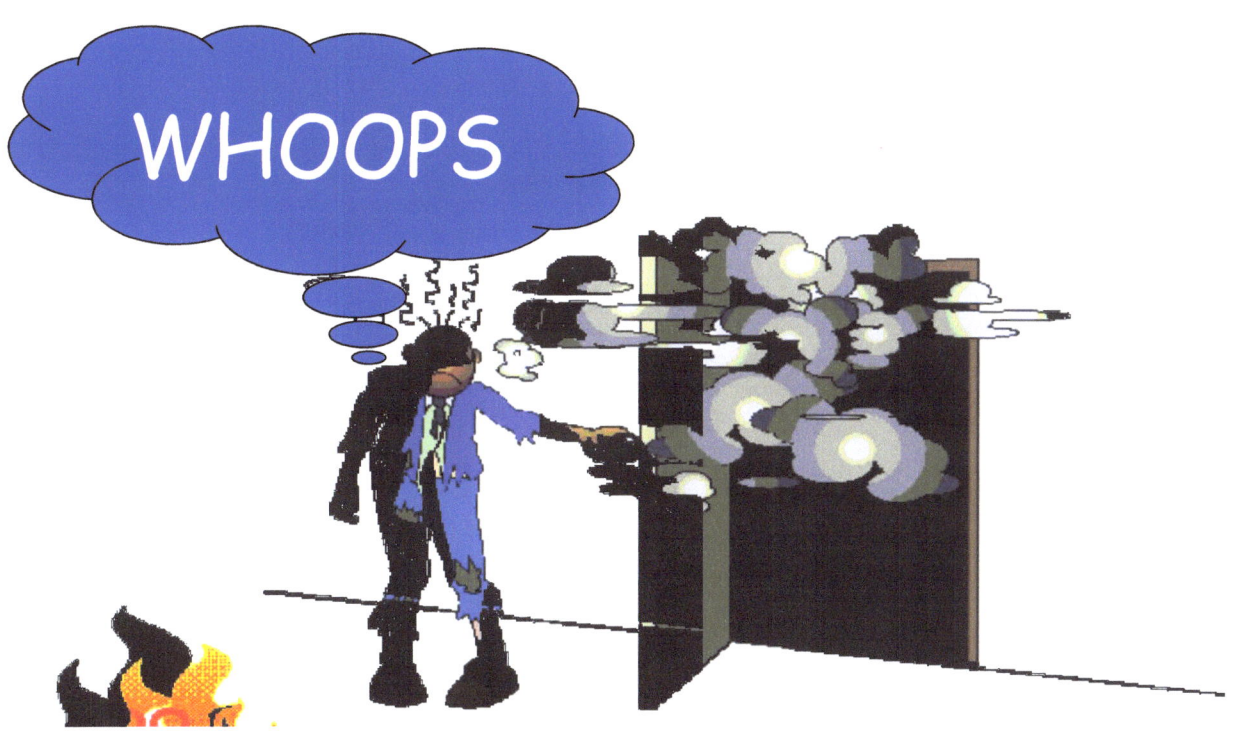

Fire Warden Kit

Mandatory in some sectors – like the care industry.

Must be easily accessible- near an entrance door.

Contents: high-vis-vest marked fire warden/marshal, a sign to direct people to the assembly point, torch, whistle, air horn, or megaphone.

If there is none in your workplace, then notify your employer.

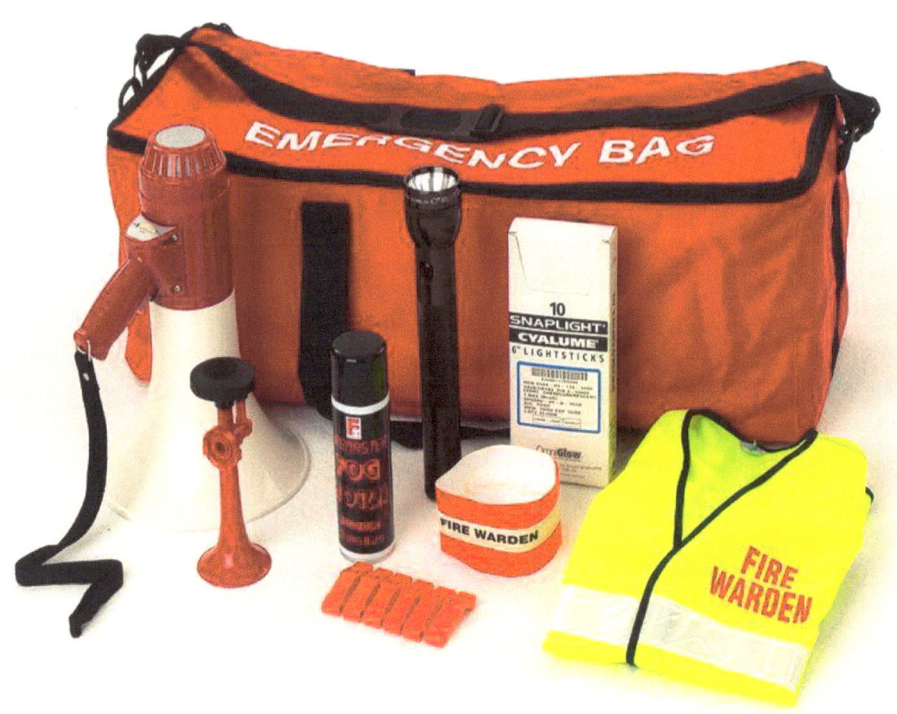

SMOKE HOODS

- This allows you to breathe as you escape from a smoke-filled room.
- They are merely used to escape through the smoke.
- Once the hood is out of the case, you place it over your head. Make sure you can breathe and leave the building.
- Once out of the building, remove the mask and breathe.

FIRE PLAN

Purpose of a Fire Plan

- To prevent fire from starting in the first place
- Prevent or minimise the loss of life in the event of a fire.
- To organise employees into teams, with each team assigned with specific tasks.
- To ensure it is confined to its origin.

Activate the alarm and ensure it is heard by all in the building and that all employees carry out their roles upon hearing the alarm activated.

Tasks to be followed.

Call the fire service.

Fight fire only if it is safe to do so.

Ensure the speedy evacuation of all employees and members of the public from the building.

Everyone must assemble at the designated assembly points.

ALLOCATION OF PERSONNEL

Where necessary, get other personnel from other parts of the complex to assist with evacuation.

Consider any special requirements- those with disabilities.

Take into consideration the special risks posed by small children and those with special disabilities who may not be able to respond quickly during evacuation.

EXERCISING THE PLAN

Employers should carry out regular fire safety exercises so that all personnel understand what their individual responsibilities are.

Employees should be aware of their individual tasks and know the building layout and any risks associated with them.

FIRE PRECAUTIONS

We can minimise or prevent fire by:

- Identifying fire hazards.
- Remove fire hazards.
- Educate staff on how to use fire extinguishers.
- Know the right fire extinguishers to use.
- Comply with emergency fire procedures.

Smoking

- Only smoke in permitted areas.
- Don't smoke where combustible materials are stored.
- Don't smoke near inflammable liquids or gases.
- Don't smoke when using aerosols.
- Don't put cigarette ends in a dustbin.
- "No smoking" areas should be properly marked.

Keep the workplace clean and tidy.

This reduces the amount of fuel for a potential fire.

Store supplies in cupboards and shelves.

Rubbish should be properly cleared.

Rubbish should be placed in metal bins with their lids on.

Regular clearance of rubbish from premises

Carry out the following routine checks on a daily, weekly, and monthly basis:

<u>Control panel checks</u>

- This will reveal when electrical alarms and fire detection systems have malfunctioned or are not working normally.
- Record any faults and deal with them.

Emergency lighting systems with signs

Make sure they are lit and malfunction is recorded.

Escape routes

Clear of obstructions

All fastenings on doors along escape routes are in working order.

All exit and directional signs can be seen clearly.

<u>Fire extinguishers:</u>

- In position
- Not discharged
- Have the correct pressure.
- And are not damaged.

FIRE DETECTION AND WARNING SYSTEMS

- They should be tested weekly for function.
- Check that it can be heard throughout the area covered.
- Ensure they can be seen and heard, especially by those with disabilities.
- Inspect and test quarterly by a nominated person.
- Inspect and test annually by a qualified engineer.
- Replaceable batteries in smoke alarms should be changed at least once a year.

BURNS AND BURNS KIT

- Run the burns under water for 20 minutes.
- Be aware of hypothermia.
- Cover with cling film.
- Follow SCALD to determine whether to take the person to the hospital.
- You can use a burn gel dressing, but it is not as effective as irrigating the burn with water.

www.ingramcontent.com/pod-product-compliance
Lightning Source LLC
Chambersburg PA
CBHW041520070526
44585CB00002B/21